WEIGHT LOSS UNLEASHED

(2024 EDITION)

Strategies for Sustainable Fat Loss

Dorothy Snow

CONTENTS

Chapter 1: Introduction   **5**

Chapter 2: Understanding the Basics   **8**

    A. Nutritional Fundamentals   8

       Caloric Deficit: 8

       Macronutrients and Their Role: 13

       Balancing Macronutrients: 15

    B. Exercise Essentials   18

       Cardiovascular Training: 18

    Strength Training   24

Chapter 3: Mindful Eating   **30**

    A. The Psychology of Eating: 30

    Understanding Emotional Eating: 30

    Breaking Free from Restriction Mindset: 36

    B. Strategies for Portion Control: 42

    C. Embracing Intuitive Eating   49

Chapter 4: Establishing Healthy Practices   **56**

    A. Developing a Sustainable Routine: 56

    B. Integration of Whole Foods: 64

    C. The Role of Hydration in Weight Loss: 66

Chapter 5: Conquering Obstacles   **70**

    A. Addressing Plateaus: 70

    B. Managing Emotional Eating: 72

    C. Sustaining Motivation: 75

Chapter 6: Embarking on Long-Term Success   **78**

    A. Lifestyle Changes vs. Short-Term Fixes: 79

    B. Building a Support System: 81

C. Celebrating Milestones:	83

Chapter 7: Tailoring Exercise Plans and Workouts 86

A. Customizing Workouts to Individual Needs:	87

B. Exemplar Workout Routines for Different Fitness Levels:	89

**Chapter 8: Nutrition Plans	94**

A. Sample Meal Plans for Various Dietary Preferences:	95

B. Cooking Tips for Healthy Eating:	100

**Chapter 9: Progress Monitoring	106**

A. Significance of Monitoring:	106

B. Technology Integration for Tracking:	109

Fitness Apps:	109

Wearable Devices:	112

Chapter 10: Sustainability Beyond Weight Metrics 123

A. Mental and Emotional Well-being:	124

B. Cultivating a Healthy Relationship with Food:	126

C. Sleep's Impact on Weight Loss:	127

**Chapter 11: Conclusion	130**

Recap of Key Strategies:	130

Encouragement for the Weight Loss Journey Ahead: 137

Chapter 1: Introduction

Welcome to "Weight Loss Unleashed: Strategies for Sustainable Fat Loss," your all-encompassing guide to establishing a healthier and enduring connection with your body. In a world saturated with quick fixes and trendy diets, this book serves as your reliable companion on the path to achieving lasting and sustainable fat loss.

In the quest for a healthier lifestyle, the focus here goes beyond the allure of swift weight loss gimmicks, exploring the importance of practices that foster long-term well-being. I will delve into how sustainable fat loss not only transforms your physical appearance but also positively influences your overall health, vitality, and mental equilibrium.

Crafting the right goals is crucial for a successful weight loss journey. "Weight Loss Unleashed" underscores the importance of setting practical and attainable objectives that resonate with your unique lifestyle and preferences. This guide will assist you in formulating goals that are not only motivating but also sustainable, ensuring a sense of achievement and ongoing progress in your fitness pursuits.

Embark on this transformative expedition with the confidence that enduring change springs from embracing sustainable strategies and setting goals that honor your individuality. "Weight Loss Unleashed" isn't merely a handbook; it represents a comprehensive approach to reclaiming your health and vigor, step by step by.

Chapter 2: Understanding the Basics

In the journey towards sustainable fat loss, gaining a clear understanding of the fundamental principles of nutrition and exercise is paramount. This chapter delves into the essential elements that form the foundation of effective weight loss strategies.

A. Nutritional Fundamentals

Caloric Deficit:

Understanding the concept of a caloric deficit is pivotal in effective weight loss strategies. This straightforward yet impactful idea revolves around the equilibrium between the calories you ingest and the calories your body expends. Here's a breakdown of its key components:

1. Energy Balance:

Your body constantly demands energy for essential functions. This energy originates from the calories present in the food and beverages you consume. Consuming more calories than your body requires results in a surplus, leading to fat storage. Conversely, consuming fewer calories than needed creates a caloric deficit, prompting your body to use stored fat for energy.

2. Fat as an Energy Reserve:

The stored fat in your body acts as a reserve for times when energy intake is insufficient. During a caloric deficit, your body taps into these fat reserves, initiating weight loss as stored fat is gradually metabolized for fuel.

3. Determining Your Caloric Needs:

It's crucial to understand your maintenance calories—the calories needed to sustain your current weight. Creating a caloric deficit involves consuming fewer calories than your maintenance level. This can be achieved through dietary adjustments, increased physical activity, or a combination of both.

4. Gradual and Sustainable Approach:

While a caloric deficit is essential for weight loss, a gradual and sustainable approach is recommended. Drastic calorie reductions can lead to nutritional deficiencies, decreased energy levels, and muscle loss. Striking a balance for steady, moderate weight loss encourages better adherence and long-term success.

5. Tracking and Adjusting:

Monitoring your caloric intake and adjusting based on progress is crucial. Keep a food diary, use apps for calorie tracking, and observe how your body responds.

Adjustments to your caloric intake may be necessary if weight loss plateaus or becomes too rapid, ensuring a consistent and sustainable progression.

In essence, a caloric deficit acts as the driving force behind weight loss. By comprehending and managing this energy balance, you wield a potent tool to shape your body composition and achieve your fat loss objectives. The key lies in finding a sustainable deficit that aligns with your individual needs while supporting overall well-being.

In the pursuit of a well-rounded and effective nutrition plan, it's essential to grasp the distinct roles of macronutrients—carbohydrates, proteins, and fats. Each macronutrient plays a specific role in supporting bodily functions and contributing to overall health.

1. **Carbohydrates**:

Carbohydrates function as the primary energy source for your body. Breaking down into glucose, they fuel essential bodily activities, including brain functions and muscle contractions. Opt for complex carbohydrates like whole grains, fruits, and vegetables for sustained energy and vital nutrients.

2. Proteins:

Proteins act as the foundational components for tissues, muscles, and organs. Consuming an adequate amount supports muscle preservation, repair, and overall growth. Additionally, protein-rich foods contribute to prolonged satiety, aiding in appetite control. Include lean meats, dairy products, legumes, and plant-based protein sources in your diet.

3. Fats:

Contrary to misconceptions, dietary fats play critical roles in the body. They contribute to hormone production, aid in the absorption of fat-soluble vitamins, and maintain cell structure. Choose healthy fats found in avocados, nuts, seeds, and olive oil while limiting saturated and trans fats from processed foods.

Balancing Macronutrients:

Achieving an optimal balance of macronutrients supports overall health and facilitates weight loss. Consider the following principles:

1. Individualized Needs:

Customize your macronutrient intake based on individual factors like age, activity level, and specific health goals.

2. Caloric Distribution:

While overall caloric intake influences weight management, how calories are distributed among macronutrients impacts body composition. A balanced distribution enhances energy levels, supports muscle maintenance, and fosters satiety.

3. Emphasis on Whole Foods:

Prioritize whole, nutrient-dense foods to ensure a comprehensive intake of macronutrients, providing essential vitamins, minerals, and fiber for overall nutritional well-being.

4. Moderation and Variety:

Adopt a varied diet that includes a moderate amount of each macronutrient. Avoid extreme approaches and fad diets to prevent nutritional imbalances and ensure long-term success.

Understanding and incorporating the functions of carbohydrates, proteins, and fats into your dietary choices not only aids your weight loss journey but also promotes overall health. Tailor your macronutrient intake to suit your unique needs, fostering a sustainable and enjoyable approach to nutrition.

B. Exercise Essentials

Cardiovascular Training:

In the realm of fitness and weight management, cardiovascular training, synonymous with aerobic exercise, emerges as a dynamic and efficient tool. This type of workout raises your heart rate and breathing, involving major muscle groups to improve cardiovascular health and play a significant role in fat loss.

1. Heart-Boosting Advantages:

Cardiovascular training is synonymous with heart health. Engaging in activities like running, cycling, swimming, or brisk walking strengthens the heart muscle, enhancing overall cardiovascular function and supporting the distribution of oxygen and nutrients throughout the body.

2. Efficient Calorie Burn:

One primary advantage of cardiovascular training for weight loss is its calorie-burning efficiency. These exercises stimulate a higher calorie expenditure, aiding in the creation of the necessary caloric deficit for shedding excess body fat. Both high-intensity interval training (HIIT) and steady-state cardio contribute to this energy expenditure, offering flexibility in workout choices.

3. Metabolic Boost Beyond Exercise:

The benefits of cardiovascular training extend beyond the workout session. Regular aerobic exercise has been shown to increase your basal metabolic rate (BMR), leading to continued calorie burning even during rest periods. This metabolic boost becomes a valuable asset in achieving and maintaining weight loss goals.

4. Enhanced Endurance and Stamina:

As cardiovascular fitness improves, so does your endurance and stamina. This means you can participate in physical activities for longer durations without fatigue. Improved stamina not only boosts overall fitness but also encourages a more active lifestyle, further contributing to weight management.

5. Versatility in Training Approaches:

The versatility of cardiovascular training lies in its various methods. Whether you opt for high-intensity interval training to elevate your heart rate or prefer steady-state cardio for a more sustained effort, there's a multitude of options to suit your preferences. Incorporating different forms of aerobic exercise keeps your routine engaging and prevents workout plateaus.

6. Holistic Health Benefits:

Beyond weight loss, cardiovascular training positively influences various aspects of health. It reduces the risk of chronic diseases like heart disease, lowers blood pressure, and improves cholesterol levels. Moreover, the release of endorphins during aerobic exercise contributes to improved mental well-being, reducing stress and enhancing mood.

To fully tap into the potential of cardiovascular training for sustainable fat loss, diversify your routine with various aerobic exercises. Whether it's a brisk morning run, an adventurous cycling session, or a refreshing swim, these activities not only aid in shedding unwanted pounds but also promote overall health and vitality. Consistency remains crucial, and finding enjoyable activities makes the journey towards your fitness goals even more gratifying.

In the realm of fitness and body transformation, strength training serves as a fundamental pillar, offering numerous advantages beyond its conventional focus on muscle development. Integrating resistance exercises into your regimen not only enhances your physical appearance but also plays a pivotal role in sustainable fat loss and overall health.

1. Metabolism Boost:

Strength training is a metabolic powerhouse, fostering the building and maintenance of lean muscle mass, contributing to an elevated basal metabolic rate (BMR). This results in increased calorie expenditure, creating a conducive environment for long-term weight management and fat loss.

2. Fat-Burning Potential:

Contrary to the notion that cardiovascular exercise is the sole fat-burning contributor, strength training plays a vital role in this process. Resistance workouts deplete glycogen stores, prompting the body to utilize fat for energy during and post-exercise. The afterburn effect, or excess post-exercise oxygen consumption (EPOC), leads to continued calorie burning after strength training.

3. Enhanced Body Composition:

Beyond weight loss, strength training sculpts and defines muscles, contributing to a leaner and more toned physique. This positive transformation in body composition influences both aesthetic goals and overall health.

4. Functional Fitness:

Strength training promotes functional fitness by improving mobility, stability, and joint health. This not only enhances your ability to perform everyday activities but also fosters an active lifestyle, supporting overall well-being.

5. Bone Health:

Building and maintaining bone density are crucial aspects of strength training. Weight-bearing exercises, including resistance workouts, stimulate bone growth and help prevent conditions like osteoporosis, particularly important with age.

6. Balanced Hormones:

Strength training positively affects hormonal balance, promoting the release of endorphins to reduce stress and enhance mood. Additionally, it contributes to the regulation of hormones associated with appetite, facilitating better control over food intake.

7. Adaptability and Variety:

Strength training provides a diverse range of exercises, allowing for adaptability and variety in your routine. From bodyweight exercises to free weights and machines, there are numerous ways to challenge your muscles, preventing workout monotony.

8. Accessible for All Fitness Levels:

Strength training is inclusive, catering to individuals of all fitness levels. Whether you're a beginner focusing on bodyweight exercises or an advanced enthusiast incorporating complex movements, the scalability of strength training accommodates diverse fitness goals.

To fully embrace the advantages of strength training for sustainable fat loss, incorporate a comprehensive resistance workout routine into your weekly schedule. Whether at the gym, at home, or outdoors, including a mix of compound and isolation exercises ensures a well-rounded approach to building strength, promoting weight loss, and enhancing overall physical well-being.

Chapter 3: Mindful Eating

In the pursuit of sustainable fat loss, cultivating a mindful approach to eating is a powerful and often overlooked strategy. This chapter delves into the psychology of eating, effective strategies for portion control, and the principles of intuitive eating.

A. The Psychology of Eating:

Understanding Emotional Eating:

Unveiling Emotional Eating: Exploring the Link Between Emotions and Food

In the intricate dance of our connection with food, emotions wield a significant influence, often steering us towards what is commonly termed emotional eating. This section delves into the subtle complexities of emotional eating, seeking to untangle its psychological intricacies and offering insights to encourage thoughtful decision-making.

1. Recognition of Emotional Triggers:

Emotional eating frequently intertwines with a spectrum of emotions, such as stress, boredom, sadness, and anxiety. The initial step in managing emotional eating patterns involves acknowledging these emotional triggers. Maintaining a journal to document instances of emotional eating can reveal patterns and provide insights into the underlying emotions associated with specific food choices.

2. The Impact of Stress:

Stress emerges as a potent driver of emotional eating for many individuals. When stress levels escalate, the inclination to seek solace in familiar, often high-calorie, foods becomes pronounced. Recognizing this connection facilitates the development of healthier coping mechanisms, such as engaging in relaxation techniques, physical activity, or mindfulness practices, to manage stress without resorting to emotional eating.

3. Addressing Boredom-Driven Eating:

Boredom frequently triggers emotional eating, prompting individuals to reach for snacks in moments of idleness. Recognizing this inclination and finding alternative activities to alleviate boredom, such as reading, taking a walk, or pursuing a hobby, can redirect the impulse to eat out of boredom.

4. Distinguishing Emotional Hunger from Physical Hunger:

Drawing a clear distinction between emotional hunger and physical hunger is pivotal. Emotional hunger tends to emerge suddenly, accompanied by specific cravings, while physical hunger develops more gradually. Taking a moment to assess the nature of hunger aids in making thoughtful decisions about whether to eat and what to eat.

5. Building Emotional Resilience:

Strengthening emotional resilience is integral to managing emotional eating. This involves cultivating coping mechanisms beyond food to navigate challenging emotions. Practices like mindfulness meditation, deep breathing exercises, or seeking support from friends and family contribute to building emotional resilience.

6. Adopting Mindful Eating Practices:

Mindful eating entails being fully present and conscious of the eating experience. When faced with emotional triggers, incorporating mindful habits—such as savoring each bite, eating without distractions, and paying attention to hunger and fullness signals—can disrupt the automatic response of turning to food in response to emotions.

Understanding emotional eating is an ongoing and dynamic process. By exploring emotional triggers, identifying patterns, and developing alternative coping strategies, individuals can break free from the cycle of emotional eating, fostering a healthier relationship with food and supporting sustainable long-term weight loss goals.

Breaking Free from Restriction Mindset:

Liberating oneself from the constraints of a rigid mindset around nutrition is a crucial step toward establishing a sustainable and positive connection with food. The inclination to impose strict dietary limitations often proves counterproductive, affecting both mental and physical well-being. This section explores the significance of breaking away from a restrictive mindset and advocates for adopting a flexible and balanced approach to nutrition.

1. Downsides of Inflexibility:

A restrictive mindset tends to foster a rigid approach to food, labeling certain items as "off-limits" or "bad." This rigid thinking can contribute to an unhealthy relationship with food, generating feelings of guilt or anxiety when deviating from predetermined dietary rules. Over time, this emotional cycle can hinder the pursuit of long-term health and weight loss goals.

2. Understanding Forbidden Food Allure:

Prohibiting specific foods can paradoxically heighten the desire for them. The attraction to forbidden foods may result in cravings and eventual overindulgence. Breaking free from the restrictive mindset involves acknowledging that all foods have a place in a balanced diet, allowing for enjoyment without guilt.

3. Adopting a Balanced Philosophy:

A balanced approach to nutrition involves viewing food as a source of nourishment, pleasure, and sustenance. Instead of fixating on rigid rules, emphasize incorporating a variety of nutrient-dense foods that contribute to overall well-being. This flexible approach fosters a more enjoyable and sustainable eating pattern.

4. Promoting Mindful Eating:

Mindful eating, rooted in being present and aware during meals, aligns with breaking free from the restrictive mindset. By relishing each bite, paying attention to hunger and fullness cues, and appreciating the sensory aspects of food, individuals can develop a healthier relationship with eating, promoting a more intuitive connection to nutritional needs.

5. Indulging Without Guilt:

Recognizing that occasional indulgences or "treat" foods are integral to a balanced diet is essential. Allowing oneself to enjoy these treats without guilt nurtures a positive relationship with food and prevents the sense of deprivation that often leads to overeating.

6. Prioritizing Nutrient Density:

Rather than fixating on calorie counting or strict meal plans, shift the focus to nutrient density. Prioritize foods rich in essential nutrients, supplying the body with the necessary fuel for optimal function. This approach accentuates the positive aspects of nutrition, fostering a sense of abundance instead of restriction.

7. Seeking Professional Advice:

For those navigating the transition from a restrictive mindset, seeking guidance from a registered dietitian or nutrition professional proves beneficial. These experts offer personalized advice, aiding individuals in establishing a balanced and sustainable approach to nutrition tailored to their unique needs and preferences.

Breaking away from a restrictive mindset signifies a liberating journey toward embracing a healthier and more positive connection with food. Through adopting a balanced approach, nurturing mindfulness in eating, and allowing flexibility in dietary choices, individuals can navigate the path to sustainable fat loss while promoting overall well-being.

B. Strategies for Portion Control:

Successfully managing portion sizes is a crucial aspect of sustainable fat loss. Implementing mindful eating techniques and adopting strategic approaches to control portions can significantly influence overall calorie intake. Here, we explore practical strategies for honing the skill of portion control.

1. Thoughtful Plate Arrangement:

Transforming your plate into a canvas for mindful eating involves intentional composition. Strive to occupy half of your plate with vibrant, nutrient-rich vegetables, allocate a quarter to lean proteins, and dedicate the remaining quarter to whole grains or healthy fats. This not only ensures a diverse nutrient profile but also naturally moderates portion sizes.

2. Opting for Smaller Tableware:

Leverage the visual impact of smaller plates and utensils. Using reduced-sized tableware creates an optical illusion of more substantial portions, promoting a feeling of satisfaction with less food. This straightforward yet effective strategy aligns with the psychology of perception, encouraging mindful consumption.

3. Appreciating Each Bite:

Embrace the practice of relishing each bite by eating slowly and intentionally. Taking the time to savor the flavors and textures of your food allows your brain to accurately register fullness. This mindful approach establishes a stronger connection to your body's hunger and satiety signals, facilitating better portion control.

4. Employing Containers and Measuring Tools:

Planning meals ahead and utilizing measuring tools, like containers or a food scale, offers a tangible way to manage portions. This proactive approach not only ensures that meals align with your nutritional goals but also removes uncertainty from portion control, empowering you to make informed decisions.

5. Hand-Based Portioning:

When specific tools are unavailable, using your hand as a guide is a practical method. For instance, a protein serving can be roughly the size of your palm, vegetables can fit into your cupped hand, and fats should be about the size of your thumb. This user-friendly technique simplifies portion control in various settings.

6. Awareness in Family-Style Dining:

Exercise mindfulness in family-style dining scenarios where large platters of food are presented at the table. This setting may encourage overeating due to the abundance of readily available food. Consider starting with smaller portions and allowing the option for seconds, promoting conscious portion control.

7. **Navigating Restaurant Portions:**

When dining out, be mindful of restaurant portion sizes, often exceeding individual dietary needs. Consider sharing dishes, opting for appetizers as main courses, or requesting a to-go box at the start of the meal to portion out a suitable amount, resisting the temptation to finish oversized servings.

8. Pre-Meal Hydration:

Drinking water before meals can instill a sense of fullness, naturally curbing your appetite and assisting in portion control. This practice not only supports overall well-being but also helps differentiate between thirst and hunger cues.

9. Embracing the 80/20 Rule:

Embrace the 80/20 rule, where 80% of your meals consist of nutrient-dense, whole foods, and 20% can include more indulgent or less nutrient-dense choices. This balanced approach allows for dietary flexibility while prioritizing health-conscious choices.

By incorporating these pragmatic strategies for portion control into your routine, you empower yourself to make mindful decisions, regulate caloric intake, and establish a sustainable foundation for successful fat loss.

C. Embracing Intuitive Eating

Intuitive eating advocates for the development of a profound connection with our bodies, encouraging a more harmonious and balanced relationship with food. Let's explore the foundational principles of intuitive eating, emphasizing a mindful and sustainable approach to nourishment.

1. Attuning to Hunger and Fullness:

Begin your intuitive eating journey by tuning in to your body's hunger and fullness cues. Instead of adhering to external schedules, learn to recognize when you're hungry and stop eating when you feel comfortably satisfied. This principle promotes a heightened awareness of your body's natural rhythms.

2. Mindful Craving Satisfaction with Nutrient-Rich Choices:

Honor and satisfy cravings with mindful choices that align with overall nutritional goals. Intuitive eating emphasizes finding nutrient-dense alternatives to indulge cravings, fostering a balanced approach that allows for enjoyment without guilt.

3. Present and Distraction-Free Eating:

Create a mindful eating environment by focusing solely on your meal without distractions. Avoid activities like watching TV or scrolling through your phone during meals to savor each bite, be present in the moment, and better recognize signals of fullness. This practice enhances the pleasure of eating and promotes conscious consumption.

4. Distinguishing Physical Hunger from Emotional Hunger:

Differentiate between physical hunger and emotional hunger, a key aspect of intuitive eating. Consider whether you are eating to nourish your body or to cope with emotions, fostering awareness and addressing emotional needs without defaulting to food.

5. Embracing Body Respect:

Integral to intuitive eating is respecting your body, appreciating its unique shape and size without succumbing to societal pressures. Developing a positive body image contributes to overall well-being and nurtures a healthy connection with food.

6. Rejecting the Diet Mindset:

Intuitive eating challenges conventional diet mentalities, advocating against restrictive cycles. Instead of external rules, it encourages an internalized approach, trusting your body's signals and fostering a sustainable, enduring relationship with food.

7. Finding Satisfaction in Eating:

Prioritize eating for satisfaction, exploring various foods and flavors to genuinely enjoy the eating experience. By savoring and deriving pleasure from meals, you enhance both physical and emotional satisfaction.

8. Cultivating Body Awareness:

Develop body awareness by paying attention to how different foods affect your body. Observe your body's responses to various nutrients and use this knowledge to inform your food choices, promoting a personalized and holistic approach to nutrition.

9. Joyful Physical Activity for Well-Being:

Engage in physical activity for the joy it brings and its positive impact on overall well-being, rather than as a mere calorie-burning endeavor. Intuitive eating encourages finding pleasure in movement, whether through structured exercise or activities that contribute to a balanced and holistic approach to health.

Incorporating these intuitive eating principles into your lifestyle empowers you to cultivate a healthier, more mindful relationship with food. This approach not only supports sustainable fat loss but also promotes overall well-being and a positive mindset toward nutrition and self-care.

Chapter 4: Establishing Healthy Practices

In the journey toward sustainable fat loss, cultivating healthy habits becomes paramount. This chapter delves into the fundamental aspects of crafting a sustainable routine, integrating whole foods, and recognizing the significance of hydration in the context of weight loss.

A. Developing a Sustainable Routine:

1. Consistency Trumps Intensity:

The bedrock of sustainable fat loss lies in consistent efforts. Instead of opting for intense but short-lived approaches, concentrate on forming habits that can be maintained over the long term. Gradual, consistent progress proves more effective than sporadic, intensive efforts.

2. Realistic and Attainable Goals:

Establishing realistic and achievable goals lays the groundwork for lasting habits. Break down weight loss objectives into smaller, manageable steps. Celebrate milestones along the way, fostering motivation for sustaining healthy habits.

3. Structured Daily Routine:

Structure serves as a scaffold for success. Devise a daily routine with designated times for meals, exercise, and rest. A well-defined schedule not only promotes discipline but also minimizes decision fatigue, facilitating adherence to healthy habits.

Crafting a daily schedule is a personalized endeavor, but here's an example routine integrating elements for overall well-being and weight loss. Adapt it based on your preferences, schedule, and individual requirements.

- **Morning:**

1. 6:30 AM - Rise and Shine:

Begin your day consistently with an early wake-up to regulate your body's natural rhythm.

2. 6:45 AM - Hydration Kickstart:

Kick off your morning with a glass of water, rehydrating your body after a night's rest.

3. 7:00 AM - Morning Workout:

Engage in a 30-minute workout, combining cardio and strength training for a metabolism boost.

4. 8:00 AM - Balanced Breakfast:

Fuel your body with a nutritious breakfast including whole grains, lean proteins, and fruits or veggies.

- **Midday:**

1. 12:00 PM - Midday Hydration and Snack:

Pause for hydration and a small, nutritious snack to maintain energy levels.

2. 1:00 PM - Wholesome Lunch:

Enjoy a lunch rich in veggies, lean proteins, and complex carbohydrates.

- **Afternoon:**

1. 3:00 PM - Afternoon Stretch or Walk:

Break up your afternoon with a brief stretch or a brisk walk to rejuvenate your body and mind.

2. 4:00 PM - Hydration and Snack:
Stay hydrated and have a small, satisfying snack to keep your energy steady.

- **Evening:**

1. 6:00 PM - Mindful Dinner:
Opt for a well-balanced dinner featuring lean proteins, veggies, and a moderate portion of whole grains.

2. 7:00 PM - Relaxation Time:
Dedicate time to relaxation activities like reading, meditation, or quality family time.

3. 8:30 PM - Unwind:

Start winding down for the night by dimming lights, minimizing screen time, and preparing for bedtime.

- **Night:**

1. 9:00 PM - Hydration and Evening Snack: If hungry, enjoy a light, healthy snack with another glass of water.

2. 9:30 PM - Bedtime Ritual: Establish a bedtime routine signaling your body it's time to wind down, such as gentle stretching or reading.

3. 10:00 PM - Rest:

Aim for 7-9 hours of sleep to support overall well-being, weight loss, and recovery.

Tailor this routine to your lifestyle, preferences, and specific needs. Add activities you enjoy and ensure it aligns with your daily commitments. Consistency is crucial, so gradually adjust and refine your routine to suit your individual goals and lifestyle.

4. Prioritize Sleep and Recovery:

Quality sleep is an often-overlooked factor in weight loss. Develop a consistent sleep routine, aiming for 7-9 hours per night. Ample rest enhances metabolic function, regulates appetite hormones, and supports overall well-being, contributing to sustainable fat loss.

1. Emphasis on Nutrient-Rich Choices:

Centralize your diet around whole, nutrient-dense foods encompassing fruits, vegetables, lean proteins, whole grains, and healthy fats. Nutrient-dense foods deliver essential vitamins and minerals, promote satiety, and contribute to overall health, making them essential for sustainable fat loss.

2. Adoption of Mindful Eating:

Foster the practice of mindful eating. Pay attention to the flavors, textures, and satiety signals of your meals. Consuming meals slowly and relishing each bite deepens your connection to the eating experience, reducing the likelihood of overindulgence.

3. Strategic Meal Preparation:

Plan and prepare meals in advance to ensure access to nutritious options throughout the week. Meal prepping not only saves time but also empowers you to make healthier choices, steering clear of the temptation of convenient yet less nutritious alternatives.

4. Limitation of Processed and Sugary Foods:

Restrict the intake of processed and sugary foods, as they frequently contribute to excessive calorie consumption. Opt for whole foods to supply sustained energy, stabilize blood sugar levels, and meet nutritional requirements conducive to sustainable fat loss.

C. The Role of Hydration in Weight Loss:

1. Prioritization of Water Intake:

Adequate hydration stands as a foundation for healthy living and weight loss. Strive to consume a minimum of 8 cups (64 ounces) of water daily. Proper hydration supports metabolic function, aids digestion, and can help regulate appetite.

2. Preference for Water Over Caloric Beverages:

Elevate water to your primary beverage choice. Sugary drinks and high-calorie beverages often contribute significantly to overall calorie intake. By opting for water, you not only effectively hydrate your body but also eliminate unnecessary empty calories from your diet.

3. Employing Hydration as a Hunger Cue:

Occasionally, feelings of hunger may be indicative of dehydration. Before reaching for a snack, consume a glass of water and wait a few minutes. Sufficient hydration can alleviate false hunger signals, contributing to your weight loss endeavors.

4. Incorporating Hydrating Foods:

Certain whole foods contribute to hydration. Include fruits and vegetables with high water content, such as watermelon, cucumber, and celery, in your diet. These foods not only hydrate but also provide essential nutrients supporting overall health.

Cultivating a sustainable routine, embracing whole foods, and recognizing the importance of hydration form the bedrock of successful and enduring fat loss. By instilling these habits, you establish a groundwork for a healthier lifestyle that extends beyond weight loss, promoting overall well-being.

Chapter 5: Conquering Obstacles

Embarking on the path to sustainable fat loss inevitably involves encountering a range of challenges. In this chapter, I'll delve into strategies to navigate and overcome common hurdles, including addressing plateaus, managing emotional eating, and sustaining motivation.

A. Addressing Plateaus:

1. Reassess Your Routine:

Plateaus are a natural part of any weight loss journey. Take a step back and evaluate your routine. Can you make adjustments to your exercise or dietary habits? Modifying your approach can kickstart progress.

2. Diversify Your Workouts:

Your body adapts to repetitive exercises, leading to plateaus. Introduce variety by incorporating new workouts or altering the intensity and duration of your current routine. This challenges your body and fosters ongoing improvement.

3. Celebrate Non-Scale Achievements:

Plateaus may not always provide a complete picture of your progress. Acknowledge non-scale victories, such as enhanced energy levels, improved sleep, or increased strength.

These indicators highlight the positive impact of your efforts beyond the scale.

4. Seek Professional Guidance:

If plateaus persist, consider consulting with a fitness trainer or nutritionist. Their expertise can offer personalized advice, helping you pinpoint specific areas that may need adjustment to overcome the plateau.

B. Managing Emotional Eating:

1. Cultivate Mindfulness:

Emotional eating often arises from a lack of awareness. Cultivate mindfulness by tuning into your emotions and recognizing hunger sensations. This mindfulness aids in distinguishing between genuine hunger and emotional triggers.

2. Establish Alternative Coping Strategies:

Identify alternative ways to cope with emotions rather than resorting to food. Engage in activities like journaling, walking, or confiding in a friend. Developing healthy outlets for emotional expression reduces dependence on food for comfort.

3. Build a Support Network:

Share your weight loss journey with friends or family who can provide support during challenging moments. A reliable support system offers encouragement and combats feelings of isolation that may contribute to emotional eating.

4. Maintain a Food Journal:

Keep a food journal to track not only what you eat but also the emotions associated with your meals. This self-awareness assists in uncovering patterns and triggers, enabling a more effective approach to addressing emotional eating.

1. Set Attainable Goals:

Define clear, achievable goals that are specific and measurable. Breaking down larger objectives into smaller, manageable milestones creates a sense of accomplishment, fueling motivation.

2. Celebrate Milestones:

Recognize and celebrate achievements along the way. Whether reaching a weight loss milestone, completing a challenging workout, or consistently making healthier food choices, acknowledging progress boosts motivation.

3. **Reconnect with Your "Why":**

Revisit the initial reasons for pursuing weight loss. Whether it's enhancing health, increasing energy, or boosting confidence, revisiting your underlying motivations reinforces commitment and rekindles motivation.

4. **Introduce Variety Into Your Routine:**

Monotony can lead to a loss of motivation. Inject diversity into your routine by trying new workouts, exploring different recipes, or incorporating various physical activities. Maintaining freshness prevents boredom and sustains enthusiasm.

5. Visualize Success:

Create a mental image of your desired outcome. Visualization serves as a potent motivator, helping you stay focused on your goals and reinforcing the belief that your efforts will lead to success.

Overcoming challenges is an integral aspect of the weight loss journey. By implementing these strategies for addressing plateaus, managing emotional eating, and sustaining motivation, you equip yourself with the tools needed to navigate obstacles and achieve sustainable fat loss.

Chapter 6: Embarking on Long-Term Success

Attaining lasting fat loss goes beyond the allure of quick fixes, requiring a comprehensive and enduring approach. This chapter immerses us in the principles of long-term success, accentuating the importance of prioritizing lifestyle changes over transient solutions. I delve into the pivotal role of constructing a resilient support system and explore the profound significance of commemorating milestones throughout the transformative weight loss journey.

1. Foster Sustainable Habits:

The essence of long-term success lies in nurturing sustainable habits that go beyond momentary fixes. Prioritize enduring changes in your lifestyle, such as embracing mindful eating, regular physical activity, and a balanced nutritional approach.

2. Transition from Diets to Sustainable Nutrition:

Depart from the constraints of restrictive diets that yield fleeting results. Embrace a nutrition plan grounded in sustainability, one that aligns with your preferences and provides a diverse array of nutrients. This approach nurtures a healthier relationship with food and underpins prolonged weight management.

3. Prioritize Consistency Over Intensity:

Opt for consistent, moderate efforts over sporadic, intense endeavors. Choose routines and practices that stand the test of time, ensuring a steady and sustainable progression toward your weight loss objectives.

1. Share Your Journey:

Constructing a robust support system emerges as a cornerstone for enduring success. Openly share your weight loss journey with friends, family, or a support group. Cultivating a network of individuals cheering you on and providing encouragement transforms the journey into a collective and manageable endeavor.

2. Seek Professional Support:

Contemplate the involvement of professionals, such as a nutritionist or fitness trainer, to guide you on this transformative journey.

Their expertise furnishes personalized advice, facilitating the navigation of challenges and ensuring a trajectory that aligns with long-term success.

3. Express Your Needs:

Establish a foundation of open communication by articulating your goals and needs to those in your support system. Whether it involves seeking understanding during challenging times or finding a reliable workout companion, transparent communication fosters an environment that nurtures support.

1. Acknowledge Non-Scale Achievements:

Beyond the numerical metrics on the scale, acknowledge and celebrate non-scale victories. Revel in increased energy levels, improved sleep quality, or heightened mental well-being. Recognizing these triumphs reinforces the positive impact of your ongoing journey.

2. Set and Celebrate Goals:

Define realistic goals and revel in their achievement. Whether conquering a fitness challenge, consistently adhering to a healthful eating plan, or attaining a specific weight milestone, commemorating these accomplishments ignites a sustained motivation for the extended journey.

3. Reflect on Progress:

Regularly carve out time for introspection, contemplating the progress you've made both physically and mentally. Acknowledge the positive changes and choices you've embraced. This reflective practice fortifies your commitment to long-term success, acting as a potent motivator for continuing the pursuit of healthful choices.

In the pursuit of sustainable fat loss, the focus shifts to the horizon of long-term success. By embracing lifestyle changes, constructing a resilient support system, and celebrating milestones, you construct a foundation for a journey that extends beyond mere weight loss to encompass comprehensive well-being.

Chapter 7: Tailoring Exercise Plans and Workouts

In the pursuit of enduring fat loss, a pivotal element involves creating exercise plans tailored to individual needs. This chapter delves into the art of customizing workouts to meet specific requirements and provides exemplar workout routines designed for diverse fitness levels.

1. Evaluate Personal Preferences:

Commence by identifying individual exercise preferences. Whether it involves outdoor activities, gym sessions, or home-based workouts, tailoring exercises to align with personal likes and dislikes enhances adherence to the fitness regimen.

2. Consider Health and Physical Conditions:

Take into account any prevailing health conditions or physical limitations. Seeking guidance from healthcare professionals or fitness experts aids in tailoring workouts that are both safe and effective, ensuring progress without compromising well-being.

3. Establish Realistic Goals:

Set achievable fitness goals based on individual starting points. Tailored workouts should challenge without overwhelming, fostering a sense of accomplishment and motivation rather than frustration.

4. Incorporate Diversity:

Ward off workout monotony by introducing a variety of exercises. Customizing routines to encompass a mix of cardiovascular, strength training, and flexibility exercises not only maintains interest but also promotes comprehensive fitness.

B. Exemplar Workout Routines for Different Fitness Levels:

- **For Beginners:**

1. Cardiovascular Exercise:

Initiate with brisk walking or low-impact aerobics for 20-30 minutes, gradually extending the duration over time.

2. Strength Training:

Integrate bodyweight exercises like squats, lunges, and push-ups. Begin with 2 sets of 10-12 repetitions.

3. Flexibility:

Include stretching exercises to enhance flexibility. Hold each stretch for 15-30 seconds, focusing on major muscle groups.

- **For Intermediate Level:**

1. Cardiovascular Exercise:

Progress to jogging or cycling for 30-45 minutes, introducing intervals for heightened intensity.

2. Strength Training:

Evolve to using weights or resistance bands for exercises such as dumbbell squats, lunges, and bench presses. Aim for 3 sets of 10-15 repetitions.

3. Flexibility and Core Work:

Expand flexibility routines and incorporate core exercises like planks and twists.

- **For Advanced Level:**

1. Cardiovascular Exercise:

Engage in high-intensity interval training (HIIT) with activities like sprints or intense cycling for 45-60 minutes.

2. Advanced Strength Training:

Integrate complex weightlifting exercises, including deadlifts, overhead presses, and advanced bodyweight movements. Target 4 sets of 8-12 repetitions.

3. Comprehensive Flexibility and Mobility:

Dedicate time to advanced stretching routines, yoga, or Pilates to enhance overall flexibility and mobility.

The crux of sustainable fat loss involves tailoring workouts to individual needs and evolving them with increasing fitness levels. By customizing exercises based on personal preferences, considering health conditions, setting realistic goals, and providing sample routines for different fitness levels, this chapter empowers individuals to embark on a fitness journey that is not only effective but also enjoyable and sustainable.

Chapter 8: Nutrition Plans

In the pursuit of sustainable fat loss, crafting effective nutrition plans is paramount. This chapter delves into the art of designing nutrition strategies that cater to various dietary preferences. It further provides practical cooking tips to facilitate healthy eating, ensuring a well-rounded and sustainable approach to weight loss.

- **Balanced Meal Plan:**

1. **Morning Meal:** Quinoa bowl with assorted berries, almonds, and a drizzle of honey.

2. **Mid-Morning Snack:** Apple slices paired with a tablespoon of almond butter.

3. **Noon Nourishment:** Grilled chicken breast, quinoa, and a medley of roasted vegetables.

4. **Afternoon Refuel:** Greek yogurt accompanied by a handful of walnuts.

5. **Evening Repast:** Baked cod with sweet potato wedges and steamed asparagus.

- **Vegetarian Meal Plan:**

1. **Breakfast Blend:** Smoothie featuring spinach, banana, almond milk, and a scoop of plant-based protein powder.

2. **Mid-Morning Snack:** Hummus alongside carrot and cucumber sticks.

3. **Lunch Delight:** Lentil and vegetable curry partnered with brown rice.

4. **Afternoon Bite:** A piece of fresh fruit, such as an orange or apple.

5. **Dinner Ensemble:** Grilled eggplant and zucchini stacks adorned with tomato

sauce and a sprinkle of nutritional yeast.

- **Low-Carb Meal Plan:**

1. **Breakfast Creation:** Omelette boasting mushrooms, spinach, and feta cheese.

2. **Mid-Morning Snack**: A handful of cherry tomatoes accompanied by mozzarella cheese.

3. **Lunch Feast:** Turkey and avocado lettuce wraps, complemented by a side of cherry tomatoes.

4. **Afternoon Munch:** Celery sticks paired with cream cheese.

5. **Dinner Harmony:** Baked salmon adorned with lemon, asparagus, and a side of sautéed kale.

- **Vegan Meal Plan:**

1. **Morning Delight:** Overnight oats crafted with almond milk, crowned with mixed berries and a sprinkle of seeds.

2. **Mid-Morning Snack:** A banana coupled with a small handful of almonds.

3. **Lunch Symphony:** Quinoa salad featuring chickpeas, cucumber, cherry tomatoes, and a zesty lemon-tahini dressing.

4. **Afternoon Savor:** Sliced bell peppers accompanied by guacamole.

5. **Dinner Fusion:** Stir-fried tofu partnered with broccoli, bell peppers, and quinoa.

These diverse meal plans underscore a rich array of nutrient-packed foods, accommodating distinct dietary preferences. Exploring these sample plans offers individuals the opportunity to find enjoyable and fulfilling ways to meet their nutritional goals, fostering a sustainable approach to weight loss.

1. Embrace Nutrient-Rich Whole Foods:

Prioritize the inclusion of whole, unprocessed foods like fresh fruits, vegetables, lean proteins, and whole grains. This foundation ensures a nutrient-dense and satisfying dietary approach.

2. Practice Mindful Portion Management:

Implement portion control to avoid overindulgence. Opt for smaller plates and bowls, and remain attuned to your body's signals of hunger and fullness, fostering mindful and balanced eating.

3. Elevate Flavors with Herbs and Spices:

Enhance the taste of your dishes without unnecessary calories by experimenting with various herbs and spices. Utilize fresh herbs, garlic, and a spectrum of spices to infuse your meals with robust and satisfying flavors.

4. Infuse Colorful Nutrient Variety:

Introduce a spectrum of colors into your meals by incorporating diverse fruits and vegetables. The vivid colors often signify a range of essential nutrients, contributing to a well-rounded and health-conscious dietary profile.

5. Restrict Added Sugars and Processed Options:

Minimize consumption of added sugars and heavily processed foods. Opt for natural sweeteners and favor whole, minimally processed alternatives, promoting a nutrient-rich and health-oriented dietary choice.

6. Strategic Meal Prep for Convenience:

Engage in planned meal preparation to ensure convenience and nutritious choices, particularly during hectic periods. Ready availability of healthful, pre-prepared meals facilitates consistency in maintaining a wholesome diet.

7. Hydration for Holistic Well-being:

Sustain proper hydration by consistently consuming water throughout the day. Adequate hydration not only supports overall well-being but also aids in distinguishing between feelings of hunger and thirst.

8. Attune to Body Signals:

Cultivate the habit of listening to your body's signals. Adopting mindful eating practices, relishing each bite, and responding to cues of hunger and fullness fosters a healthier relationship with food, encouraging a balanced and sustainable eating pattern.

9. Incorporate Lean Protein Sources:

Prioritize lean protein choices such as poultry, fish, tofu, and legumes. These protein-rich selections contribute to a sense of fullness and assist in preserving muscle mass during weight loss.

10. Diversify Cooking Techniques:

Explore various cooking methods such as grilling, baking, steaming, and sautéing. This diversity not only introduces variety to your meals but also allows for experimentation with different flavors and textures.

By tailoring sample meal plans to various dietary preferences and providing practical cooking tips, this chapter equips individuals with the tools to create sustainable and enjoyable nutrition plans on their weight loss journey.

Integrating these culinary strategies into your routine not only enhances the nutritional value of your meals but also transforms the act of healthy eating into an enjoyable and sustainable endeavor. Embrace creativity in the kitchen to discover a plethora of delicious and health-conscious culinary options.

Chapter 9: Progress Monitoring

Embarking on the path to sustainable fat loss requires a systematic approach to evaluating and tracking your journey. This chapter underscores the importance of monitoring progress and explores the integration of technology for effective and streamlined tracking methods.

A. Significance of Monitoring:

1. Alignment with Goals:

Consistent monitoring ensures that your actions align with your weight loss objectives.

By keeping tabs on your progress, you can pinpoint areas of success and those requiring adjustments, ensuring steady progress towards your desired outcomes.

2. Behavioral Insight:

Monitoring extends beyond numerical data, fostering awareness of your behaviors. Understanding the impact of your habits on your progress empowers you to make informed decisions, cultivating sustainable behavioral changes contributing to long-term fat loss.

3. Motivation and Responsibility:

Tangible progress serves as a potent motivator. Whether it's measurable changes in body dimensions, enhanced fitness levels, or positive shifts in health markers, tracking achievements boosts motivation and holds you responsible for your weight loss journey.

4. Pattern Recognition:

Monitoring enables you to discern patterns in your eating, exercise, and lifestyle habits. Identifying these patterns, whether advantageous or challenging, provides valuable insights for refining your approach and overcoming obstacles.

1. Fitness Applications and Wearables:

Harness the capabilities of fitness apps and wearable devices to track physical activity, monitor workouts, and analyze trends. These tools offer real-time feedback, providing a comprehensive overview of your fitness progression.

Fitness Apps:

1. MyFitnessPal:
    - Characteristics: Tracks calories, logs food, monitors exercises, and provides community support.

- Available on: iOS, Android.

2. Nike Training Club:

    - Attributes: Offers personalized workouts, guides exercises through videos, and tracks progress.

    - Available on: iOS, Android.

3. Strava:

    - Features: GPS tracking for running and cycling, social connectivity, and analysis of performance.

    - Available on: iOS, Android.

4. Fitbod:

   o Characteristics: Tailors workout
     plans, adapts training, and tracks
     progress.

   o Available on: iOS, Android.

5. MapMyRun:

   o Features: GPS tracking, route
     planning, and detailed workout
     analysis for running.

   o Available on: iOS, Android.

6. 7 Minute Workout:

   o Attributes: Quick, intense

     workouts for time-efficient

     exercise.

   o Available on: iOS, Android.

Wearable Devices:

1. Fitbit:
   o Features: Tracks activity,

     monitors heart rate, analyzes

     sleep, and sets goals.

   o Examples: Fitbit Charge, Fitbit

     Versa, Fitbit Sense.

2. Apple Watch:

- o Features: Fitness tracking, heart rate monitoring, ECG, GPS, and a variety of health apps.

  - o Examples: Apple Watch Series 6, Apple Watch SE.

3. Garmin:

  - o Characteristics: GPS sports watches with activity tracking, heart rate monitoring, and performance analytics.

  - o Examples: Garmin Forerunner series, Garmin Venu.

4. Samsung Galaxy Fit:

    o   Features: Tracks fitness and sleep, monitors heart rate, and provides notifications.

    o   Example: Samsung Galaxy Fit 2.

5. Xiaomi Mi Band:

    o   Attributes: Budget-friendly fitness trackers with heart rate monitoring, sleep tracking, and activity monitoring.

    o   Examples: Xiaomi Mi Band 6.

6. Whoop Strap:

   o   Characteristics: Tracks strain,
       optimizes sleep, and monitors
       recovery.

   o   Example: Whoop Strap 4.0.

These applications and wearable devices offer
a variety of functionalities to suit different
fitness objectives, preferences, and financial
considerations.

2. Nutrition Tracking Apps:

Employ nutrition tracking apps to log your
daily food consumption. These apps often
include extensive databases with nutritional

information, helping you stay aware of calorie intake, macronutrient balance, and overall dietary habits.

EXAMPLES

1. MyFitnessPal:

Characteristics: Monitors calories, macronutrients, and micronutrients with an extensive food database and barcode scanning.

Platform: Available on iOS and Android.

2. Lose It!:

Attributes: Tracks food consumption, establishes personalized goals, and facilitates easy input with a barcode scanner.

Platform: Available on iOS and Android.

3. Cronometer:

Features: Specializes in tracking micronutrients and provides comprehensive information on the nutritional content of foods.

Platform: Available on iOS and Android.

4. Yazio:

Characteristics: Monitors calories, macronutrients, and exercise, offering personalized meal plans and recipes.

Platform: Available on iOS and Android.

5. SparkPeople:

Features: Tracks food intake, exercise, and water consumption, incorporating goal-setting features.

Platform: Available on iOS and Android.

.

6. MyPlate by Livestrong:

Attributes: Tracks calories, macronutrients, and exercise, with a focus on weight loss and healthy eating.

Platform: Available on iOS and Android.

7. Carb Manager:

Features: Specializes in tracking carbohydrate intake, making it suitable for low-carb and keto diets.

Platform: Available on iOS and Android.

8. FatSecret:

Characteristics: Tracks food intake, exercise, and weight, with a community for sharing progress and recipes.

Platform: Available on iOS and Android.

9. MyNetDiary:

Features: Monitors calories, macronutrients, and exercise, with additional features for diabetes management.

Platform: Available on iOS and Android.

10. Eat This Much:

Attributes: Generates meal plans based on dietary preferences, tracks food intake, and provides recipes.

Platform: Available on iOS and Android.

These apps provide diverse features to assist users in tracking their nutrition, achieving dietary goals, and making informed choices about their food intake

3. Smart Scales and Body Composition Monitors:

Integrate smart scales and body composition monitors for a holistic perspective on your progress. Beyond weight, these devices offer insights into body fat percentage, muscle mass, and hydration levels, providing a more comprehensive understanding of changes.

4. Online Communities and Support Networks:

Engage in online communities and support groups to share progress, challenges, and triumphs. The communal aspect fosters encouragement, accountability, and opportunities to learn from individuals on similar journeys.

5. Regular Consultations with Professionals:

Schedule periodic check-ins with healthcare professionals or fitness experts. These experts can offer personalized guidance, assess progress, and provide recommendations tailored to your individual needs and goals.

6. Journaling and Reflection:

Merge technological tools with the traditional practice of journaling. Reflecting on experiences, emotions, and challenges provides a holistic perspective on your weight loss journey, promoting mindfulness and self-awareness.

In conclusion, monitoring progress stands as a dynamic and essential element of sustainable fat loss. By grasping the importance of monitoring, embracing technology for tracking, and utilizing a variety of tools and methods, you empower yourself to navigate your journey with insight, motivation, and adaptability.

Chapter 10: Sustainability Beyond Weight Metrics

Attaining sustainable fat loss encompasses more than numerical indicators on the scale. This chapter delves into key factors crucial for enduring success, placing emphasis on mental and emotional well-being, nurturing a positive connection with food, and recognizing the pivotal role that sleep plays in the weight loss journey.

1. Mindful Consciousness:

Foster mindful awareness of thoughts and emotions, acknowledging the multidimensional nature of the weight loss journey. Regular self-reflection enhances comprehension of one's relationship with the body and the holistic aspects of the weight loss process.

2. Positive Affirmations:

Cultivate positive self-talk and celebrate victories beyond physical changes. Recognizing achievements like increased energy, improved mood, and enhanced confidence contributes to a sustainable and gratifying weight loss experience.

3. Stress Management Practices:

Integrate stress management practices, including meditation, deep breathing exercises, or yoga. Recognizing the impact of chronic stress on weight loss efforts, incorporating relaxation techniques supports mental well-being and overall health.

1. Intuitive Eating Approaches:

Embrace intuitive eating by attuning to your body's hunger and fullness signals. Avoid strict dietary rules and restrictions, fostering a balanced and enduring approach to food. This mindful connection with the body promotes healthier eating habits.

2. Diversity and Enjoyment in Nutrition:

Prioritize a diverse and enjoyable array of foods, incorporating nutrient-rich choices and emphasizing the pleasure of each meal. A varied and pleasurable diet enhances satisfaction, reducing the likelihood of feelings of deprivation.

3. Balanced Indulgences:

Allow occasional indulgences without guilt, recognizing that moderation is key. Treating yourself on occasion is a part of a balanced lifestyle, eliminating the notion of "forbidden" foods and minimizing the risk of binge-eating tendencies.

C. Sleep's Impact on Weight Loss:

1. Establishing Healthy Sleep Patterns:

Prioritize consistent and quality sleep by establishing a routine that promotes restful nights. Acknowledge the connection between inadequate sleep and disrupted metabolism, understanding that quality sleep enhances overall well-being and supports weight loss.

2. Understanding Hormonal Influence: Recognize the influence of sleep on hormonal balance, particularly with hormones like leptin and ghrelin that regulate appetite. Quality sleep contributes to a healthier hormonal profile, reducing cravings and the likelihood of overeating.

3. Stress Alleviation Through Sleep: Consider sleep as an essential aspect of stress reduction. Quality sleep aids in managing

stress levels, indirectly supporting weight loss by minimizing stress-induced cravings and emotional eating.

In essence, sustainable fat loss goes beyond numerical benchmarks. By prioritizing mental and emotional well-being, fostering a positive relationship with food, and acknowledging the significance of quality sleep, individuals lay the foundation for a comprehensive and enduring approach to weight loss.

Chapter 11: Conclusion

As we wrap up this exploration into sustainable fat loss, let's revisit the pivotal strategies that form the bedrock of lasting success. Furthermore, let this concluding chapter be a wellspring of encouragement for the thrilling journey ahead in your pursuit of weight loss.

Recap of Key Strategies:

1. Caloric Deficit Unveiled:

- Grasping the pivotal role of a caloric deficit as the cornerstone for weight loss.

- Embracing mindful eating and portion control as essential components in achieving and sustaining a caloric deficit.

2. Macronutrients and Their Significance:

- Understanding the importance of macronutrients – proteins, fats, and carbohydrates – in crafting a balanced and enduring diet.

- Tailoring macronutrient intake to individual preferences and needs.

3. Cardiovascular Training:

- Incorporating cardiovascular training as an effective means for burning calories and enhancing overall cardiovascular health.

- Balancing cardio exercises with diverse physical activities for a comprehensive fitness regimen.

4. Strength Training:

- Acknowledging the benefits of strength training in building lean muscle, elevating metabolism, and improving overall body composition.

- Integrating strength workouts into the fitness routine for sustained health gains.

5. Mindful Eating Insights:

- Delving into the psychology of eating and adopting strategies for cultivating mindfulness and intuition in dietary habits.

- Confronting and overcoming emotional eating patterns for enduring progress.

6. Building Healthy Habits:

- Establishing a sustainable routine that incorporates whole foods, emphasizes hydration, and integrates mindful habits into daily life.

- Recognizing the impact of hydration on weight loss and overall well-being.

7. Overcoming Obstacles:

- Navigating plateaus, managing emotional eating, and maintaining motivation throughout the weight loss journey.

- Strategies for liberating oneself from a restrictive mindset and fostering a positive connection with food.

8. Long-Term Triumph:

- Discerning the distinction between lifestyle changes and transient fixes for a comprehensive approach to health.

- Cultivating a support system and commemorating milestones as integral elements of enduring success.

9. Tailored Exercise Plans:

- Customizing workouts to individual needs, considering fitness levels and preferences.

- Presenting sample workout routines for various levels to inspire diversity and consistency.

10. Nutrition Plans:

- Offering sample meal plans for diverse dietary preferences, promoting variety and enjoyment.

- Providing cooking tips for healthy eating, encouraging ingenuity and mindful food choices.

11.   Progress Monitoring:

- Acknowledging the significance of tracking progress for goal alignment, behavioral awareness, and motivation.

- Leveraging technology for efficient progress tracking, incorporating fitness apps, nutrition tracking apps, and smart devices.

12.   Sustainability Beyond the Scale:

- Prioritizing mental and emotional well-being, fostering a positive relationship with food, and understanding the role of sleep in weight loss.

- Embracing a holistic approach that extends beyond numerical achievements to ensure lasting success.

Encouragement for the Weight Loss Journey Ahead:

As you embark on your personal weight loss narrative, remember that this journey is exclusively yours. Every stride, regardless of its size, is a triumph. Embrace the journey, stay committed to your objectives, and extend kindness to yourself throughout. Sustainable fat loss transcends the transformation of your body; it encompasses the evolution of your lifestyle and the nurturing of a healthier, more fulfilled version of yourself.

Challenges may arise along the way, but armed with the strategies you've acquired, you possess the means to overcome them. Each health-conscious decision, every conquered workout, and each mindful bite contributes to a more resilient, vibrant you.

As this chapter concludes and you step into the next segment of your journey, may you find delight in the pursuit of health, strength in facing challenges, and an unwavering belief in your ability to achieve sustainable fat loss. Your journey is a testament to your fortitude and determination – an unbridled odyssey with the promise of a brighter, healthier tomorrow.

www.ingramcontent.com/pod-product-compliance
Lightning Source LLC
Chambersburg PA
CBHW070845260726
48661CB00004B/1251